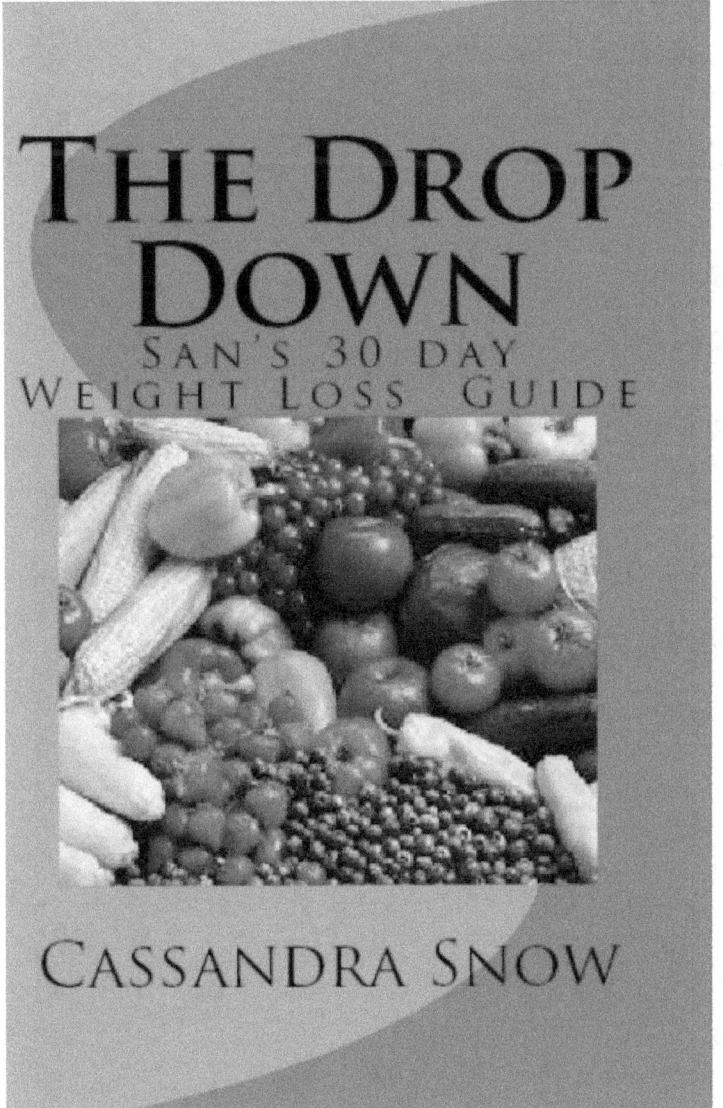

THE DROP DOWN

SAN'S 30 DAY
WEIGHT LOSS GUIDE

CASSANDRA SNOW

Contents

Dedication

I dedicate this book to my family, friends, and everyone struggling with weight loss and health issues. To all of the naturopaths and healers who have enlightened me on my way. To my beautiful children who always believe in me no matter what, and for putting up with me when I went cold turkey on my journey to wellness. And most importantly to God for your undying love, and for supplying every need every day in every way.

Peace, Love, Good Health and Blessings to you all

Your Mentor, Your Sister, Your Family, Your Mother, Your Friend

Cassandra D. Snow

Introduction

Throughout the years I've realized that the key to achieving optimal health is not through pills, shakes, and liquid potions, but by the renewing of your mind, and by choosing the foods God has given us to sustain perfect health.

The body is comprised of many cells that if damaged can be renewed by the foods we choose to put in it. In this guide I share my health journey with you, and provide you a jump start into a new way of how to look at food, a list of healthy foods to eat, and a thirty day food plan to get you on the right track to optimal health.

This guide can be used over and over again if needed, but it is my hope that after your first thirty days you will be inclined to continue on your journey to perfect health, and never look back.

My very best thoughts to you on your new journey!

Health Declaration

I declare God's continued blessings over my life, and my health.

I am a perfect image of God, and I will see an outburst of God's will for me to obtain perfect health. I will experience the weight loss and optimal health I have desired for so long. I will choose to feel good, and put only good things in my body at all times. My body is my temple, and my temple is comprised of nothing but the best foods and nutrition. My perfect body is on its way. This is my declaration.

NOW   THEN

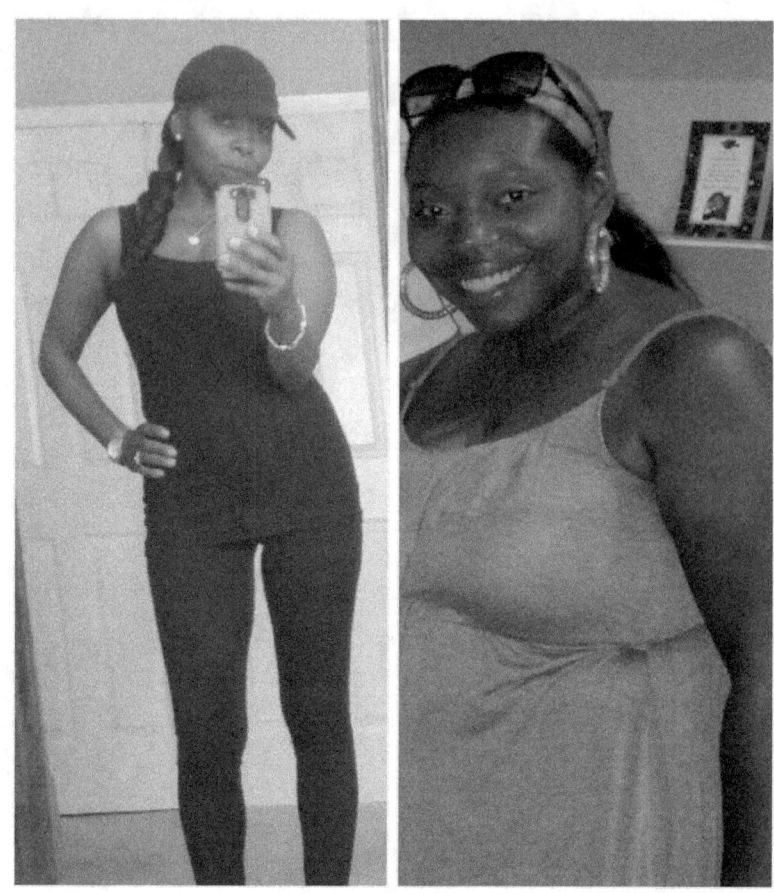

Chapter 1

My Story! The health crisis that started it all

In 1998 I began to encounter serious ophthalmic headaches, bringing on unbearable pain to my eyes and head. Subsequent to consulting with several Retina and Cornea Specialists and having many tests taken for them all to return negative, and to be informed this was an interminable condition. I came to the realization this could be a condition I would have to live with for the rest of my life.

During this medical crisis and due to the mix of various meds, stress, and an unhealthy eating regime; I began gaining weight. During my life and even after bearing children I had managed to keep my weight under control, but noticed my body was slowly coming to an unhealthy state. During my health crisis, I had become solely dependent on pain medications specifically in the mornings just to start my day. The pain I endured in my eyes and head in the mornings were unbearable, hence me starting my day with 800 mg ibuprofen every day for nearly a year.

A year and a half had nearly gone by with dealing with all the tests, and stress, and pain, and a friend who knew of my illness approached me with a body cleansing and detoxifying product. They stated that it had helped people lose weight, cleanse their bodies, and just jump start them into better health. Inside the packet of what was called a five day cleanse had a total of six pills in them. It included herbs like Psyllium, Black Walnut, Cascara Sagrada, Iris moss, and many more products designed to cleanse and detoxify the body. On the third day of using these products I noticed that I woke up with no headache and a burst of energy but more importantly I eliminated more waste than I could ever remember in my entire life. After all I had gone through, and enduring this pain daily, waking up with this feeling was extremely amazing and very exciting!

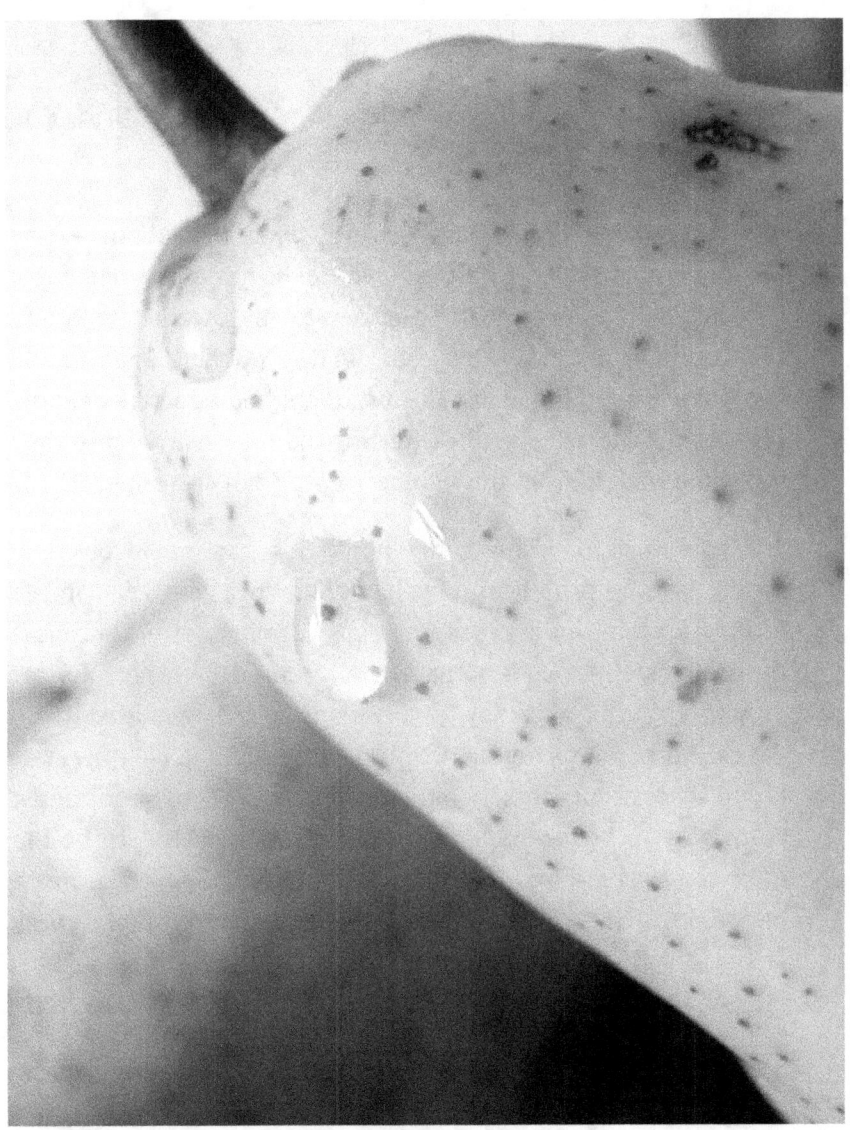

Pears-Eating whole pears are excellent for its precious fiber, and are highly beneficial for your colon health. The pectin in pears is a diuretic and has a mild laxative effect. Drinking pear juice regularly helps regulate bowel movements which are ideal for assisting in weight loss.

Chapter 2

The Wellness Journey Begins! Thank God for optimism

Although I had always been pretty conscious about eating healthy and intrigued by alternative medicines and procedures. I wasn't conscious enough to use it to my own personal life consistently until now. Because I felt so good I began to tell everyone around me about this product I had been taking, how wonderful I was feeling, and referring them to my friend so they too could benefit from this wonderful world of cleansing.

Subsequently, me sharing my outcomes got me involved in promoting the products as well. During this time I became a product of the product. Not only was I feeling better, but I lost three dress sizes, built a team, and created extra income for myself. To think a packet of six cleansing pills would start an entire journey into better health. I was fully enjoying my new found success, business, health and wellness. More importantly, I was able to help others do the same. I found this to be the most rewarding thing of all. Just to hear people say how much better they felt, or how much weight they lost was very pleasurable to me.

I would have healthy home parties, travel to support others, and attend national conventions. I was enjoying this healthy lifestyle journey. Then my life took a drastic turn!

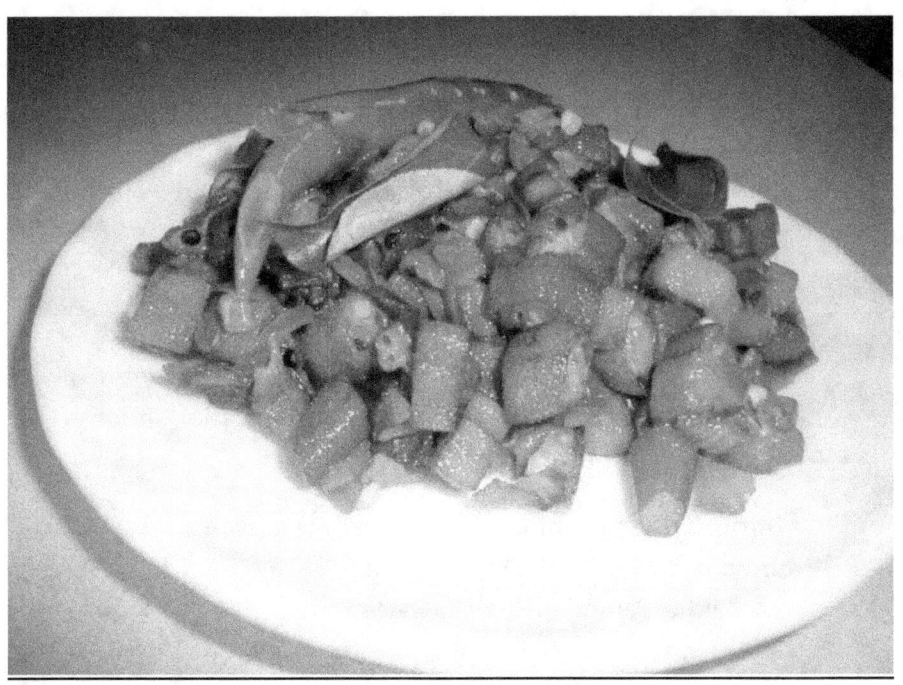

Okra- Okra includes rich sources of dietary fiber, minerals and vitamins, and is highly recommended in controlling weight. Okra also contains healthy amounts of vitamin A and flavonoid anti-oxidants. They are also rich in B-complex group of vitamins like vitamin B6. They also contain good amounts of vitamin K. Okra is also a good source in minerals such as iron, calcium and magnesium.

Chapter 3

Embracing Change! Change is good.

Several years had gone by; it was now 2005, although I wasn't promoting the products as much as the previous two years. I was still marketing them part time, staying as healthy as I could, and encouraging others to do the same.

During this time I found myself dealing with an awful separation, unfortunate divorce, and relocation from NJ to Atlanta GA within a matter of months.

Throughout this unforeseen life changing event, I experienced some of the most challenging times of my life. I found myself unhealthy, emotionally challenged, and financially drained. After going through this roller coaster ride of first losing weight during this stressful time, I also began to slowly gain weight. My eating habits had become poor; I was drinking alcohol, partying regularly, and not exercising. These bad habits continued for several years. In between those challenging times because of my previous experience with network marketing, I had been introduced to several weight loss, and health and nutrition programs of which I tried the products and also marketed several of them; some of which were really great products in their own way but did not offer me the health and nutrition I found with fasting, and eating foods that provide optimal health.

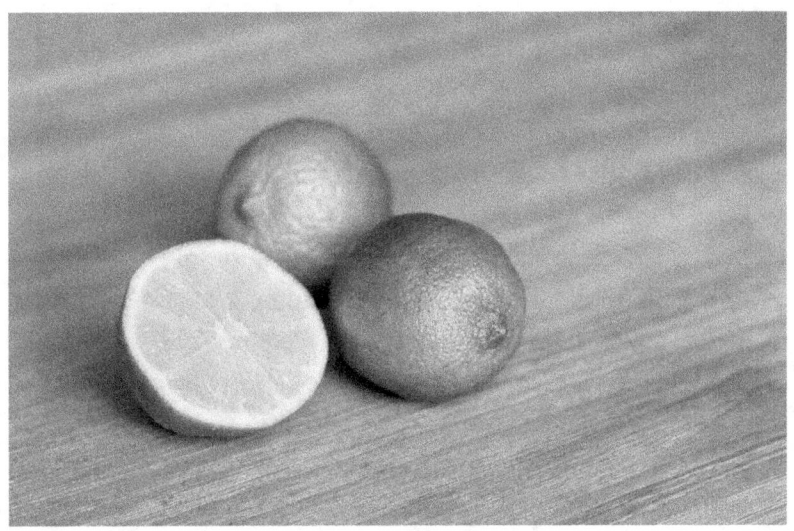

Limes-Limes have been proven to help with eye care, weight loss, skin care, improve digestion, and respiratory disorders. Limes are an excellent source of vitamin C, B6 and potassium. Limes may also help the prevention of diseases such as heart disease, and the hardening of arteries.

Chapter 4

My light bulb moment

After several trips to the doctor and knowing my weight, several looks in the mirror, and a denial of not being able to fit in certain clothing; it wasn't until the summer of 2014 that I realized something drastic had to be done. I took a long hard look at some of the pictures I was featured in that summer, and realized I was spiraling out of control. Here I was a health conscious woman, conscious of what to eat, what to do, how to do it, and I wasn't doing it. I was ashamed of myself! I was so ashamed that although vowed not to get involved in another marketing company, I sought out a weight loss product that involved a cleansing product, and daily shakes. Although this product afforded me a temporary fix on feeling good and losing weight; I found myself becoming dependent on using these products to keep my weight off, and began to put the pounds back on.

A year later I came across a Holistic Dr. discussing the benefits of being a Vegan and the health benefits it provides. Although I had known the health benefits of eliminating certain foods from one's diet and encouraging others to do the same. I had never thought of how important the quote from Hippocrates "Let food is thy medicine and medicine is thy food." really was. Something clicked, THIS WAS IT! I instantly realized that if I wanted to achieve long lasting optimal health for the rest of my life. It wasn't going to come from shakes and pills, but from a total lifestyle change. A change that was going to require lots of research on the healthiest foods, mental and physical strength, a resistance to temptations, and perseverance. I studied and researched for weeks day in and day out and finally decided I was going to do it! I was going to try out this new found lifestyle. I was going to test this totally vegan diet out just to see what results I could achieve. I immediately went cold turkey, stopped eating all animal products, and focused strictly only on fasting, eating only fruits, vegetables, and drinking spring water. Within thirty days I had unbelievably lost twenty six pounds and felt the best I had felt in years. I couldn't believe it, I had literally lost five pounds a week with no exercise, no shakes, no pills, but with a healthy group of fruits and vegetables compiled by me through trial and error, and pairing foods to my liking.

It was then I discovered I had something. I had something that not only worked, but worked quickly, and I had to share! For years I had been encouraging people to lose weight and adopting a healthier lifestyle, but I realized I had been doing it all wrong. I had been encouraging people to put ingredients in their bodies that I nor them could even pronounce when in reality everything a person needs to become leaner and healthier comes from God and is right in your garden, grocery store, and or farmers market.

It is why I decided to share my journey, and this thirty day guide to catapult you into a leaner body, and a healthier way of how you look at what you put into your bodies. It is why I bring to you "The Drop Down". I hope this guide provides you the power to take control of your health, to love yourself more, and achieve the results you have desired for so long. I love you all and may God bless you on your journey!

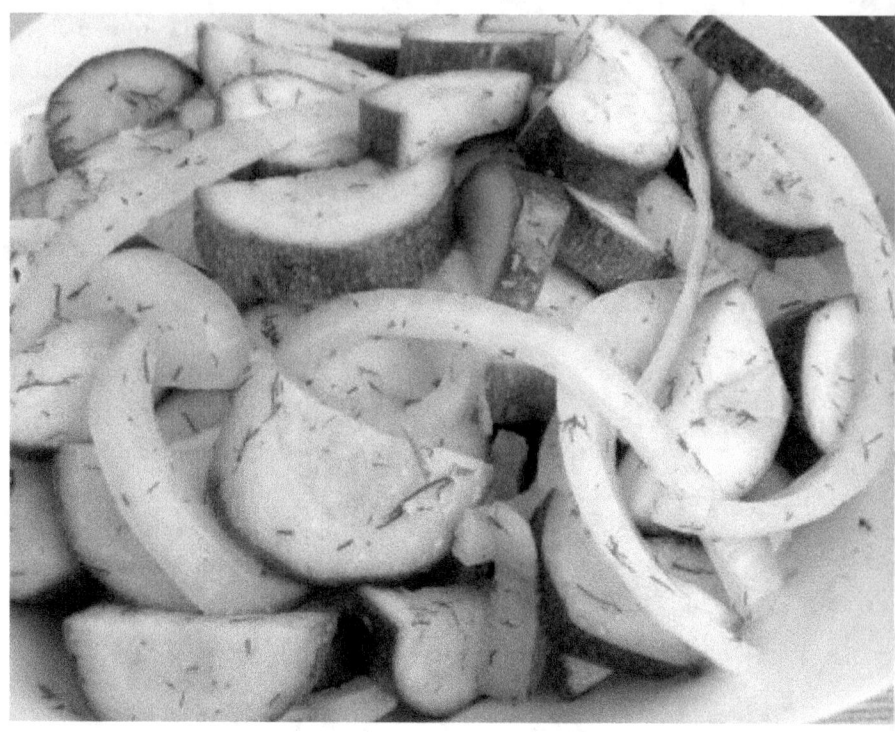

Zucchini - Zucchini is well known for reducing weight, and boosting valuable nutrients. Zucchini promotes eye health, and has a high content of vitamin C. Zucchini is a great way to make you feel fuller, and is a great way to satisfy appetites. It is also a great source of dietary fiber.

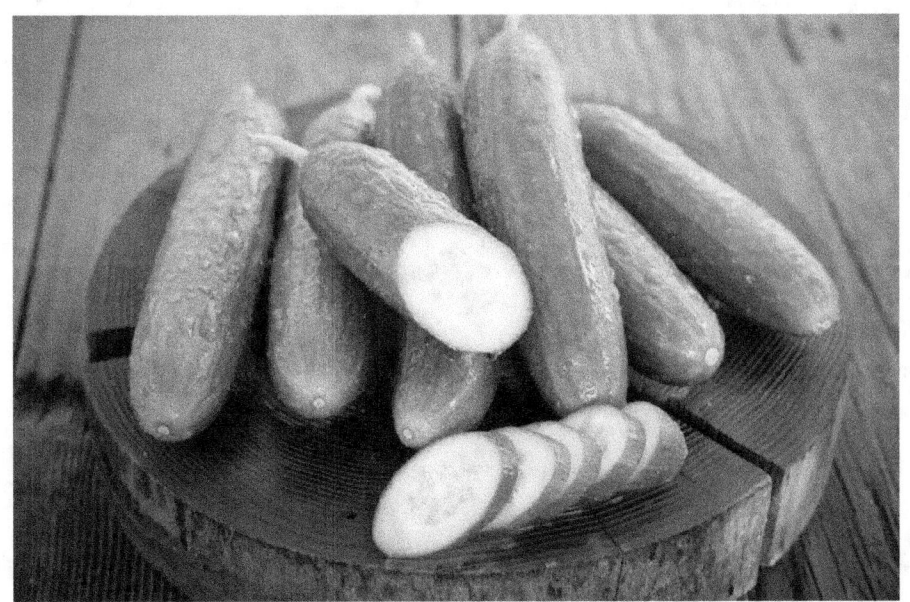

Cucumbers – Cucumbers are great for flushing out toxins, aiding in weight loss, cutting cancer, reviving the eyes, keeping you hydrated, and supplying the body with vitamins, minerals, magnesium, and potassium. Cucumbers also help protect the brain, fights inflammation, and support the digestive system.

Chapter 5

"The Guide"

San's 30 Day weight Loss Guide to never worry about your weight Again!

You may use this guide as often as you need to achieve your desired weight loss goals. The foods listed in this guide are all alkaline nontoxic foods that will heal you, and help you obtain optimal health.

The foods you will need throughout your 30 days:

- Spring Water
- Apple, Pear, or Orange Juice
- Lime Juice
- Ginger Tea
- Raspberry Tea
- Kale
- Turnip Greens
- Yellow Squash
- Butternut Squash
- Zucchini
- Plum/Cherry Tomatoes
- Sun Dried Tomatoes
- Cucumbers
- Onions
- Bell Peppers
- Baby Bella or Portabella Mushrooms
- Parsley
- Avocados
- Romaine Lettuce
- Other Lettuce if desired (No iceberg)
- Okra
- Olives (Green or Black)
- Garbanzo/Chick Peas
- Limes
- Green Apples,

- Seeded grapes
- Red Apples
- Mango's
- Cantaloupe
- Small Bananas (Preferably Burro Mini Bananas)
- Papayas
- Walnuts
- Raisins
- Dates (optional)
- Sea salt
- Onion power
- Cayenne Pepper
- Ground Ginger
- Sesame Oil
- Grape seed Oil
- Spelt or Rye Bread
- Quinoa or Rye Pasta
- "Black" wild rice

Week 1

What you will need:

- Kale
- Green Apples
- Small Bananas (Preferably Burro
- Limes
- Avocados
- Romaine Lettuce
- Cucumbers
- Tomatoes (optional)
- Parsley
- Onions
- Bell Peppers
- Okra (optional)
- Turnip Greens
- Sesame Oil
- Grape seed oil (optional)
- Sea Salt
- Onion Powder
- Pure Agave Nectar
- Spring Water
- 100% Pure Non concentrated Pear or Apple juice
- Coconut Milk
- Lime Juice

Day 1-2 Fast no solid foods (8-10 8 oz. cups spring water with lime, three 4 oz. servings of non-concentrated 100% pure pear juice or apple juice) *Either of these juices is ok.

Day 3-7 You will eat the following every day during these days for Breakfast, Lunch, and Dinner

 Breakfast- 1 cup Kale, ½ green apple, 1 cup coconut milk, 1tbsp agave nectar, 1 small banana or 2 Burro bananas (mini bananas)

Lunch 1 sliced avocado, 2 cups romaine lettuce, 1 cucumber, (key lime juice, sea salt, agave nectar, cayenne pepper, avocado oil or grape seed oil, onion powder for taste) Combine ingredients to create a healthy salad.

Or you may use tomato, cucumber, onion, parsley as an alternate.

Dinner- 1 lb. Turnip greens, 1 medium onion, 1 green bell pepper. Slice onion, and pepper. Sauté all the ingredients with sesame oil, season with sea salt and onion powder until brown, simmer for 20 min or until desired consistency.

Or you may have tomatoes, mushrooms, onions, bell peppers, okra, and sautéed in sesame oil or grape seed oil.

Week 2

What you will need:

- Limes
- Papayas
- Romaine Lettuce
- Squash
- Zucchini
- Cucumbers
- Plum or Cherry Tomatoes
- Parsley
- Onions
- Bell Peppers
- Baby Bella or Portabella Mushrooms
- Okra (optional)
- Turnip Greens
- Olives (Green or Black)
- Sesame Oil
- Grape seed oil (optional)
- Sea Salt
- Onion Powder
- Pure Agave Nectar
- Spring Water
- 100% Pure Non concentrated Pear or Apple juice
- Coconut Milk
- Lime Juice

Day 1 -5 You will eat the following every day during this time for Breakfast, Lunch, and Dinner

Breakfast- ½ papaya, ½ cup coconut milk or 1 cup depending on desired consistency, 1 tbsp. agave nectar, ice, blend in blender. (Ice optional)

Lunch- 1 sliced cucumber, 1 serving of sliced plum or cherry tomatoes, 2 cups romaine lettuce, ½ cup olives black or green. (Lime juice, olive oil, sea salt as desired) Combine ingredients to create a delicious healthy salad.

Or you may use tomato, cucumber, onion, and parsley as an alternate.

Dinner- 1 sliced squash, 1 sliced zucchini, ½ onion ½ green bell pepper, 1 cup portabella or baby bella mushrooms, sautéed in sesame oil. Sautee ingredients in sesame or grape seed oil, simmer 15 min or until desired consistency

Or you may have tomatoes, mushrooms, onions, green peppers, okra, and sautéed in sesame oil or grape seed oil.

Day 6-7 Fast no solid foods (8-10 8 oz cups spring water with lime, three 4 oz. servings of non-concentrated 100% pure pear, apple or orange juice) *Either of these juices is ok.

Week 3

What you will need:

- Spring Water
- Apple, Pear, or Orange Juice
- Lime Juice
- Kale
- Sun Dried Tomatoes
- Onions
- Bell Peppers
- Romaine Lettuce
- Other Lettuce if desired (No iceberg)
- Limes
- Green Apples,
- Seeded grapes
- Red Apples
- Mango's
- Cantaloupe
- Small Bananas (Preferably Burro Mini Bananas)
- Walnuts
- Raisins
- Dates (optional)
- Garbanzo/Chick peas
- Spelt or Rye Bread
- Pure Agave Nectar
- Sea salt
- Ground Ginger
- Onion power
- Cayenne Pepper
- Sesame Oil
- Grape seed Oil
- Spelt or Rye Bread

Day 1-5 You will eat the following every day during this time for Breakfast, Lunch, and Dinner

Breakfast - 1 small sliced organic apple, 1 small banana (preferably mini burro banana) 1 piece of spelt (bread) or 100% rye bread toast, you may spread on raw agave nectar for taste. You may drink Ginger or raspberry tea. 1 tsp Agave nectar can be added for flavor

Or you may have 1 serving of sliced cantaloupe, 1 slice of Spelt or 100% rye toast spread with raw agave nectar. Ginger or Raspberry tea. 1 tsp of Agave nectar for taste.

Lunch – 2 cups of any lettuce of your choice (except iceberg) 1/2 mango sliced, 1 cup walnuts, 1 cup apples, ½ cup dates or seeded raisins. Combine ingredients, you may add sea salt and lime for flavor as desired

You can rotate with – Any lettuce (except iceberg) apples, seeded grapes, walnuts, seeded raisins.

Dinner –1 jar 8oz Sun dried tomatoes chopped, ½ lb. of kale, 1 can Garbanzo/Chick peas, 1 can coconut milk, 1 small onion, sea salt, onion powder , cayenne pepper, ground ginger, agave nectar as desired. Heat oil in a large deep skillet over medium-high heat. Add onion and cook for about 5 minutes. Add Sun-dried tomatoes, and cayenne pepper.

Cook for approx. 5 minutes, stirring frequently. Add the chickpeas and cook over high heat until golden. Add in kale, stir and wait for it to cook down. Pour in the coconut milk, sea salt, ground ginger cayenne pepper, Bring to a simmer, then turn down the heat and cook for 10 minutes. Taste and add more seasonings as desired.

Day 6-7 - Fast no solid foods (8-10 8 oz. cups spring water with lime, three 4 oz. servings of non-concentrated 100% pure pear juice or apple juice) *Either of these juices is ok.

Week 4

What you will need:

- Spring Water
- Apple, Pear, or Orange Juice
- Lime Juice
- Butternut Squash Soup
- Parsley
- Kale
- Onions
- Other Lettuce if desired (No iceberg)
- Baby Bella or Portabella Mushrooms
- Limes
- Red Apples
- Mango's
- Small Bananas (Preferably Burro Mini Bananas)
- Quinoa or Rye Pasta
- "Black" wild rice (optional)
- Coconut Milk
- Pure Agave Nectar
- Sea salt
- Ground Ginger
- Onion power
- Cayenne Pepper
- Sesame Oil
- Grape seed Oil
- Spelt or Rye Bread

Day 1-5 You will eat the following every day during this time for Breakfast, Lunch, and Dinner

Breakfast – Kale, banana, mango, coconut milk. Combine 1 cup chopped Kale, ½ cup coconut milk, 1 small banana, ½ cup sliced mango 1tsp of Agave nectar. Combine all ingredients in a blender on high until smooth.

Lunch – 8 oz. of Butternut squash soup, 1 serving of chopped parsley. (You may purchase a 32 oz. carton of Organic Butternut squash soup)

Dinner- 1 serving of either Quinoa or Rye pasta, ½ onion, ½ bell peppers, ½ cup baby bella or portabella mushrooms, cayenne pepper, sea salt, onion powder, Agave nectar (optional) as desired. Sautee onion peppers and mushrooms to desired consistency. Serve over cooked pasta.

Or you may alternate with a serving of wild black rice and a serving of sautéed turnip greens and onion.

Day 6-7 - Fast no solid foods (8-10 8 oz. cups spring water with lime, three 4 oz. servings of non-concentrated 100% pure pear juice or apple juice) *Either of these juices is ok.

Important tips to remember

- Do no drink alcohol or caffeine
- Do not substitute the Agave Nectar for ANY other sweeteners
- Drink 70 ounces of water per day as your body is made of 70% water. This is roughly 8-10 glasses per day
- If you get extremely hungry during fasting you may have seeded watermelon or cantaloupe
- Do not eat meat, fish, or chicken. (This guide is based on a Vegan Diet) The more alkaline your body becomes, the faster you will start to heal and lose weight
- Take your fasting days very seriously. Fasting is very powerful! Fasting helps the body heal the body, removes toxins, and reduces stress and inflammation.
- Keep a positive attitude. If you think you can you will!
- Contact me with any questions or concerns about any of the food items, alternatives, or where you can find them
- Always consult with a health care provider before attempting any weight loss plan
- Stay away from negative people. This is your journey!
- You are a powerful human being! Focus only on the results you want to achieve and not the pain you may endure while achieving them.
- I believe in you! Believe in yourself!

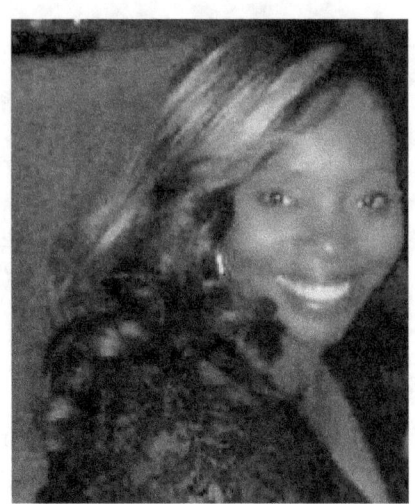

About the Author

Cassandra Snow aka "San" is a Health and Wellness Consultant who is on a journey to lead millions of people to optimal health. Cassandra's compassion for helping people, and more importantly her desire for everyone to achieve healthier fulfilled lives in every area, makes her a pivotal leader in helping others reach their wellness goals. Cassandra's caring heart and easy way of communicating provides a refreshing journey into health and wellness. Outside of that Cassandra enjoys spending fun times with her four children, Isis, Emil, Elijah, and Emanuel. The Drop Down is Cassandra's first guide to health and wellness.

Connect with Cassandra via

Facebook - https://www.facebook.com/sansnowenterprises/

Instagram - https://www.instagram.com/sansnow.co/

Email – csnowenterprises@gmail.com